中医药文化故事

（汉英双语）

Stories of Traditional Chinese Medicine Culture
(In Chinese & English)

金　虹　王晓珊　陈岷婕　／主编
高剑坤　邹　微

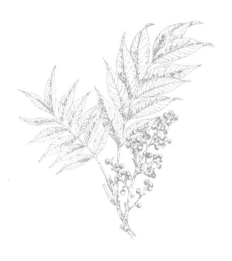

四川科学技术出版社

图书在版编目（CIP）数据

中医药文化故事：汉、英 / 金虹等主编. -- 成都：
四川科学技术出版社, 2023.8
　　ISBN 978-7-5727-1115-2

　　Ⅰ. ①中… Ⅱ. ①金… Ⅲ. ①中国医药学—文化—汉、
英 Ⅳ. ①R2-05

中国国家版本馆CIP数据核字(2023)第146624号

ZHONGYIYAO WENHUA GUSHI (HANYING SHUANGYU)

中医药文化故事（汉英双语）

主编 金虹　王晓珊　陈岷婕　高剑坤　邹微

出 品 人	程佳月
策划组稿	钱丹凝
责任编辑	税萌成
封面设计	墨创文化
封面题字	汪涌泉
版式设计	大　路
责任出版	欧晓春
出版发行	四川科学技术出版社
地　　址	四川省成都市锦江区三色路238号新华之星A座25层
	传真：028-86361756　邮政编码：610023
成品尺寸	130 mm × 185 mm
印　　张	2.75　字　数 55 千
印　　刷	四川华龙印务有限公司
版　　次	2023年8月第 1 版
印　　次	2023年9月第 1 次印刷
定　　价	29.00元

ISBN 978-7-5727-1115-2

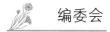 编委会

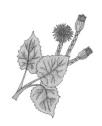

前言

　　中医药具有浓厚的中国传统文化色彩，融合了中国哲学包含的儒家、道家和佛家思想，是中华优秀传统文化重要的组成部分。几千年来，中医药对中华民族的生存繁衍、疾病防治和强身健体发挥了重要作用。习近平总书记指出"中医药学是中国古代科学的瑰宝，也是打开中华文明宝库的钥匙"。《中医药文化故事（汉英双语）》作为四川省高校中华优秀传统文化重点建设课程的组成部分，采用汉英双语的编写形式，旨在通过一些中医药方面的小故事，讲解其中蕴含的历史文化背景知识，让更多的人了解博大精深的传统中医，同时在充分认识中国传统文化的基础上，更好地弘扬中医药文化。

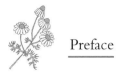 Preface

Deeply rooted in Traditional Chinese Culture, Traditional Chinese Medicine (TCM) integrates many philosophical ideas from Confucianism, Taoism and Buddhism, and it continues to be an important element of Chinese culture. For thousands of years, traditional Chinese medicine has played an important role in the survival and reproduction of the Chinese nation, disease prevention and control, as well as physical fitness. General Secretary Xi Jinping points out that "Chinese medicine is not only the treasure of ancient Chinese science, but also the key to opening the treasure house of ancient Chinese civilization". As an integrated part of the key construction course contents of excellent traditional Chinese culture in colleges and universities of Sichuan province, compiled in both Chinese and English, *Stories of Traditional Chinese Medicine Culture* aims to explain some historical and cultural background knowledge behind traditional Chinese medicine through selected short stories, so that more people can understand the extent and profundity of traditional Chinese medicine. The culture of traditional Chinese medicine could therefore be carried forward, based on a fuller understanding of traditional Chinese culture.

目录
CONTENTS

第一章　著名医家的故事

Section One　Stories of Famous Physicians

中华上下五千年，在这漫漫的历史长河中，涌现出了许多中医药大家。从神医扁鹊到药王孙思邈，从华佗到李时珍，从医圣张仲景到金元四大家，他们大医精诚所表现的高尚医德和成就，永远激励后辈守正创新，继往开来。

　　Chinese history have existed for 5,000 years. In this long history, many Chinese medicine masters have emerged, from Bian Que, a miracle doctor, to Sun Simiao, known as the king of medicine; from Hua Tuo to Li Shizhen; from Zhang Zhongjing, a medical sage, to the four masters in the Jin and Yuan Dynasties. With noble medical ethics and great achievement, they have always inspired successors to remain upright and innovative, as well as carry forward our medical cause and forge ahead into the future.

药王孙思邈 "大医精诚"

Sun Simiao: a Great Doctor with Proficient
Medical Skills and Exalted Medical Ethics

辛夷花

在四川省绵阳市北川县，有一个盛产中药材的地方叫"药王谷"。每年春天，漫山遍野的辛夷花吸引着来自全国各地的观光游客。在山顶有一尊高大雄伟的药王孙思邈的塑像，药王谷因此而得名。

In Beichuan county, Mianyang city, Sichuan province, the Yaowang Valley region abounds in herbs. Each spring, the magnolia flowers that bloom throughout the mountains attract visitors from all over the country. On top of the mountain stands a majestic statue of Yaowang (the King of Medicine) Sun Simiao. Thus, the Yaowang Valley is named after Yaowang Sun Simiao.

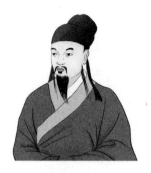

孙思邈

　　孙思邈（581–682），隋唐时期陕西铜川人。自幼多病，为筹医药费，几乎用尽家财。这促使他萌生了学医的想法。他从 18 岁起便潜心研究中医，熟读百家学说，20 岁便通晓医药知识，包括儿科、内科、外科以及五官科，尤其擅长针灸、按摩与食疗。他在编撰的《千金要方》中提出"大医精诚"的中医药核心价值观，其中"人命之重，有贵千金，一方济之，德逾于此"强调了医学执业者应德艺双馨，这句话也成为中国医学生的入行誓言。

Sun Simiao (581—682 A.D.) was born in Tongchuan city, Shanxi province, and lived during the Sui and Tang Dynasties. When he was a child, he was constantly ill. To cover medical expenditures, his family's wealth was nearly depleted, which prompted him to study medicine. He had devoted himself to the study of Traditional Chinese Medicine from the age of 18, meticulously and repeatedly reading hundreds of medical theories. By the time he was twenty, he possessed a thorough grasp of medicine, including paediatrics, internal medicine, surgery, and otolaryngology. Additionally, he excelled at acupuncture, massage, and dietary therapy. In his book *Qian Jin Yao Fang* [*Prescriptions Worth a Thousand Pieces of Gold*], he proposed that mastership of medicine lies in proficient medical skills and exalted medical ethic, which eventually became core values that have been conscientiously upheld by the TCM field. He pointed out that "Human life is of paramount importance, more precious than a thousand pieces of gold, and one prescription which can save it is even more precious.", this phrase highlighted the combination of virtue and skills needed by medical practitioners and became the oath of medical students.

传说，孙思邈在行医途中遇见了抬棺者抬着一口棺材，后面还跟着一个年轻人和一对老夫妻。孙思邈得知棺材内是年轻人的妻子，因难产而"死"，遂仔细观察，发现棺材下的血还是鲜红色的，就大声要求打开棺材，看是否能救人一命。开棺之后发现该女子面色苍白，但尚有一丝脉搏，孙思邈迅速取出银针，对准穴位扎下去，不久该女子的心跳恢复了，并产下一名婴儿，全家人都惊呆了，对孙思邈的救命之恩感激不尽。

According to legend, on his way to practice medicine one day, Sun Simiao encountered pallbearers carrying a coffin, followed by a young man and an elderly couple. Sun Simiao attentively inspected the coffin after learning that the young man's wife had died in childbirth, noticing that the blood beneath the coffin was a vivid red. To save a life, he yelled for the coffin to be opened. After this had been done, Sun Simiao discovered the woman inside was pale but still had a feeble pulse. He drew out a silver needle and inserted it rapidly into an acupuncture point. Soon afterwards, the woman's heart rate returned to normal and she gave birth to a healthy baby. The entire family was astonished and highly appreciative of Sun Simiao's assistance.

　　孙思邈在他一百岁高龄的时候，还完成了《千金要方》的补充《千金翼方》，方中记载了800多味药材和2000余个古方。"凡药皆须采之有时日"强调采药季节的重要性，列举了233种药物的采制时间，熟地黄"九蒸九晒"的炮制方法也流传至今。他是对药物的保管提出"药藏"的第一位医家，为古代药物学发展作出了巨大贡献。此外，孙思邈还创立了养生十三法，如"发常梳""目常运""齿常叩"等，提出养生的核心在于养

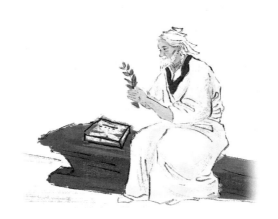

性，主张淡泊名利、生活简朴。

When he was one hundred years old, Sun Simiao also compiled *Qian Jin Yi Fang*, a supplement to *Qian Jin Yao Fang* [*Invaluable Prescriptions for Emergencies*], in which more than 800 medicinal herbs and more than 2,000 ancient prescriptions were recorded. He stated, "Every herb must be gathered for a specific length of time", underlining the critical nature of the herbal harvesting season. In the book, he listed the harvesting time for 233 different herbs and the "nine steaming and nine drying" method of cooking rehmannia, which has been handed down until modern times. He was the first physician to propose a "medicine collection" for the storage of herbs, making a major contribution to the development of ancient pharmacology. In addition, Sun Simiao also established 13 health preservation practices, such as "combing your hair frequently", "turning your eyes regularly", and "clicking your teeth consistently". He proposed that the essence of health maintenance lay in cultivation of nature and advocated a simple lifestyle free from the desire for fame and fortune.

神农尝百草
Shen Nong Undertook Trials of Hundreds of Herbs

　　相传神农是厉山氏的儿子，也称炎帝，他平日里教导人们伐木农耕。由于不忍心看到人们因吃错食物而中毒，神农发誓要尝遍各种草本植物并加以记载。他左右肩各挎一个草药袋，每当他尝到治病的草药时就放在右边的袋子里，而普通的可食用的草就放在左边袋子里。在这一过程中，神农也会不小心吃到有毒的东西，便积极寻找服用可以解毒的草药，并把有毒的植物记载下来警告人们不要服用。

　　According to legend, Shen Nong was the son of the Lishan Clan, also known as the Yan Emperor, who taught people how to cut logs and cultivate in their ordinary days. Not wishing to see people poisoned by eating the improper food, Shen Nong vowed to taste and record various plants.

with a bag on each shoulder, he placed therapeutic herbs in the bag on the right whenever he tasted them, while placed plain edible grass in the bag on the left. During this process, Shen Nong would also accidentally eat poisonous substances, so he would actively look for herbal medicines that could detoxify him before writing down the poisonous plants to warn other not to use them.

　　不幸的是，神农误服了一种叫"断肠草"的植物，还没来得及服用解毒药，断肠草的毒性就发作了，神农也就永远地离开了人世。断肠草，其实就是中药"钩吻"，有显著的镇痛和催眠作用，但也具有毒性。"神农尝百草，始有医药"的故事，也是今天大家耳熟能详的"药食同源"的来历。神农对祖国医学的探索和献身精神一代又一代地流传下来，他也被后世称为"医药之祖"。

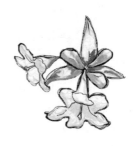

钩吻（断肠草）

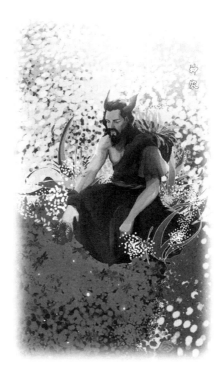

神农尝百草

Unfortunately, Shen Nong accidentally ingested a plant called "heart-broken grass". Before he could take the antidote, the plant's poison erupted and Shen Nong passed away. In fact, "heart-broken grass" is, also known as "gelsemium" in traditional Chinese medicine, which possesses significant analgesic and hypnotic properties, as well as a high potential for toxicity. Since Shen Nong tasted all types of plants, this legend of Chinese medicine began to spread. The well-known "medicine and food homology" also originated from this story. Shen Nong was also known as the "Father of Medicine" due to his exploration and devotion to Chinese medicine, which has passed down from generation to generation.

神医扁鹊的故事
The Story of Bian Que,
a Miracle-Working Doctor

在春秋战国时期，还是孩子的扁鹊拜名医长桑君为师，扁鹊留在长桑君的医馆里刻苦钻研医术。有一日，长桑君外出采药，两个年轻人抬着一位老奶奶进来求医，扁鹊还是学徒，不敢看病，但是看到老奶奶病情危急，便试着按了按老奶奶的穴位，并诊脉开了药方抓了药给老奶奶。没想到年轻

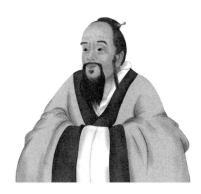

神医扁鹊

人不小心将药包摔破在木匠铺前，年轻人也没钱重新买药，只好就地抓起药来抱回了家。长桑君外出回来之后听了此事经过，审查了药方，发现扁鹊少加了一味檀香在药里，这样很可能让老奶奶服药无效病重而死。正在扁鹊要去追回药的时候，年轻人和老奶奶来感谢扁鹊的救命之恩。长桑君和扁鹊一问，才知道年轻人将木匠铺地上的木头渣子一起捡起来熬药了，那木头渣子正好是所缺的檀香木。

During the Spring and Autumn and Warring States Periods, Bian Que, although still a child, learned medical knowledge form Chang Sangjun, a famous doctor. He stayed at Chang's clinic and studied medical skills assiduously. One day, when Chang went out to gather herbs, two young people came in carrying an old woman and seeking a doctor. Bian Que, as an apprentice, dared not treat the patient. However, seeing the grandmother's critical condition, he tried to press her acupoints, feel her pulse and prescribe medicine for her. Unexpectedly, the young man accidentally shattered the herbs bag in front of the carpenter's shop. As he had no money to buy new medicine, the young man was forced to pick up the herbs to carry them home. After returning and discovering the situation, Chang Sangjun reviewed the prescription and found that Bian Que had omitted sandalwoods from the medication, a mistake which was likely to aggravate the grandmother's condition to the point of death. When Bian Que was about to retrieve the medicine, the young people and the grandma came to thank Bian Que for saving her life. Making inquiries, Chang Sangjun and Bian Que discovered that the young man had cooked the medicine together with the wood residue left on the ground by the carpenter, which happened to be the missing ingredient, sandalwood.

　　从那时开始，扁鹊谨记老师教诲，看病抓药都非常谨慎，因为他知道中医配方讲究协同搭配，或多或少、哪怕错一味都会影响到治病的效果甚至关系人命。渐渐地，他的医术远近闻名，名气越来越大，他给民众带来了健康，由于医术高超，人们借用《黄帝八十一难经》的著者"神医扁鹊"来称呼他。

Thereafter, Bian Que kept his tutor's teachings in mind and was highly cautious when treating patients and writing prescriptions. Bian Que was aware that the TCM formula emphasised coordination and collocation, so the dosage and accuracy of each herb affected the healing and even the lives of individuals. Gradually, he became well-known throughout the world for his excellent medical skills. Since he brought health to the people, he was named "Magical Doctor Bian Que" after the author of *Huang Di Ba Shi Yi Nan Jing* [*The Eighty-one Classics on the Medical Problems of the Yellow Emperor*].

第二章　神奇的针灸历史与文化

Section Two　Acupuncture Therapy's Mystical History and

Culture

2017 年 1 月，国家主席习近平在瑞士日内瓦访问，他向世界卫生组织赠送了一尊针灸铜人作为国礼，吸引了全世界的目光。针灸起源最早可追溯到新石器时代，人们在生活劳作中常常会发生风湿和创伤性疼痛，就会自然地以揉、捏、捶、击打加上火烤来除湿和缓解疼痛。石块是最常用的一种，因此逐渐产生了以"砭石"（又称针石）为工具的医疗方法。灸法是在人类发现火之后，原始人将烧热的石块用于缓解身体某部位的疼痛所形成热熨法，这两者被视作针灸的萌芽。后经不断地探索改进和演变，银针取代了砭石，艾草燃烧温熏替代了石块热熨，针刺和艾灸合起来形成了我们现在常说的针灸疗法。

In January, 2017, Chinese President Xi Jinping visited Geneva, Switzerland, where he presented a bronze acupuncture figure to the World Health Organization as a national gift, capturing the world's attention. Acupuncture therapy may date from the Neolithic Period. During their everyday job routines, people frequently suffered from rheumatism and acute pain. To dehumidify and ease their discomfort, people in the past instinctively turned to kneading, pinching, hammering, beating, and even moderate heat treatment. The most commonly used tool was stone. As a result, a medical treatment utilising a "stone", also referred to as a "stone needle", eventually developed and gained widespread acceptance. Moxibustion was invented in response to the emergence of fire. Historically, humans used heated pebbles to alleviate physical discomfort, which was the birth of acupuncture with moxibustion. Metal needles eventually supplanted stone needles, while burning or heating dry wormwood supplanted warm stones. Acupuncture and moxibustion combined to form the acupuncture therapy that is now familiar.

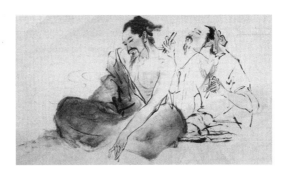

2000 多年的医疗实践经验表明，单独使用针灸治疗的疾病可有 80 多种， 配合其他疗法能治疗的疾病有 500 多种。1972 年， 美国总统尼克松访华的时候，随行记者莱斯顿在北京协和医院接受针灸治疗，此事在《纽约时报》头版进行了报道，随后世界范围内掀起了针灸热潮，并在美国 44 个州合法化。许多国家开设了针灸相关医学课程，并激发更多人对这一神奇的传统医学疗法产生了浓厚的兴趣。2010 年， 中医疗法针灸入选联合国教科文组织人类非物质文化遗产代表作名录。

Over 2,000 years of medical practice experience has demonstrated that acupuncture can cure more than 80 diseases independently and more than 500 disorders when coupled with other therapies. In 1972, during President Richard Nixon's visit to China, an accompanying reporter, Richard Reston, received acupuncture treatment at Peking Union Medical College Hospital. This was reported on the front page of the *New York Times*, sparking a worldwide acupuncture craze and leading to its legalisation in 44 US states. Numerous nations have developed acupuncture therapy schools and public interest has been widely aroused. Acupuncture and moxibustion therapy were included on the 2010 UNESCO Intangible Cultural Heritage of Humanity list.

王惟一与针灸铜人
Wang Weiyi and Bronze Acupuncture Figures

  在北宋初期，针灸非常盛行，可是关于针灸的古籍却有错讹。这时，著名的医家，身为宋仁宗和宋英宗御医的王惟一，主管医疗教学和医疗考试，精于针灸的他受到了寺庙里大佛铜像的启发，认为如果能够铸造一具铜像，上面准确地刻上经络与穴位，岂不是能规范针灸教学与考试吗？于是他多次上书皇帝请求考证针灸之法并铸造针灸铜人作为针灸之准则，并反复设计铜像草图，精打细磨，费了一番周折最终将草图与构想一并呈给皇帝。

Acupuncture therapy was quite popular throughout the early Northern Song Dynasty. However, older texts on acupuncture and moxibustion lacked precision. The renowned acupuncture doctor Wang Weiyi worked for two emperors, Song Renzong and Song Yingzong, and was in charge of medical teaching and inspections. He was inspired and enlightened at the time by a bronze statue of Buddha in a temple. Given his skills in acupuncture, he confidently reasoned that if a bronze figure could be made with exact engravings of meridians and acupoints, would not it be feasible to standardise acupuncture education and examinations? As a result, he wrote to the emperor on many occasions, pleading to verify acupuncture's therapeutic techniques and construct bronze figures to standardise the acupuncture and moxibustion principles and acupoints. He redesigned the bronze statue several times, attempting to perfect every aspect. Finally, after considerable effort, he submitted his ideas and design sketches to the emperor.

终于，功夫不负有心人，在天圣五年（1027 年），王惟一奉宋仁宗之命，负责设计并主持铸造了两具针灸铜人，从塑胚到铸造完成他都全部亲力亲为。两具针灸铜人均仿制成年男子身形而制成， 躯壳前后由两件构成，内置脏腑，外刻腧穴。各穴位与体内相通，外涂黄蜡，内部灌水，如刺中穴位，则液体溢出，若稍有偏差，针则不能刺入。这样，针灸铜人就可以作为医生经穴试针和教学考试的工具。两具针灸铜人犹如精湛的艺术品一样受到了宋仁宗的夸赞，便下令保留一具模型供太医院教学之用，另一具置于大相国寺内供人观摩。

Finally, his efforts were rewarded. Emperor Song Renzong tasked Wang Weiyi to cast two bronze acupuncture figures in the fifth year of Tiansheng (1027 A.D.). He completed the casting himself, from moulding to finish. The two bronze figures were formed into the shape and size of mature young men. The torsos were made of two parts, with internal organs and acupoints engraved on the front and back. Each acupoint was wired internally. Water was infused into the interior and yellow wax was added to the exterior, which acted similarly to human skin in covering and concealing the acupoints. When specific acupoints were penetrated, the liquid flowed out; if it did not, the needle had not pierced the correct spot. As a result, the bronze acupuncture figures were used to educate, perform, and examine acupuncture. The emperor lavished admiration on the two beautiful bronze statues, which resembled works of art. He directed that one be kept for education and the other be put in the Great Temple for public worship and admiration.

同时，王惟一还整理编撰了《铜人腧穴针灸图经》配合铜人使用。在这一过程中，他把很多不统一的针灸学著作加以去伪存真。同时，他以铜人为式，分脏腑十二经，旁注腧穴，将十二经脉，三百五十四个穴位，直观地描绘下来，并对前代经穴学说进行了订正，推动了中国针灸学的发展。最重要的是，王惟一针灸铜人的发明，促进了经穴教学的形象化与直观化，并开创了针灸腧穴考试实操的先河。

At the same time, Wang Weiyi also compiled a book, *Tong Ren Shu Xue Zhen Jiu Tu Jing* [*Illustrated Manual of Acupoints on a Bronze Figure*], to complement the use of the bronze figure. By doing so, he preserved the truth by expunging several contradictory publications on acupuncture and moxibustion. He divided the viscera into 12 meridians by using the bronze statues as models and labelled the acupoints by name on the side. Thus, 12 meridians and 354 acupoints were shown plainly and methodically. Additionally, he reviewed and refined the existing literature on acupuncture and moxibustion, significantly accelerating the development of acupuncture theories and practice. Most significantly, the creation of the bronze figures provided a visual representation of the meridian and acupoint instructions, and established a precedent for the practical application of acupuncture and moxibustion exams.

宋代以后，人们又陆续制造了一些针灸铜人。遗憾的是，这些铜人几乎都在战乱中损毁，那两尊宋代制造的铜人也至今下落不明。

Following the Song Dynasty, additional identical bronze figures for acupuncture teaching were gradually created. Regrettably, nearly all were destroyed by war. The two bronze figures made in the song Dynasty remain lost and unidentified to this day.

针灸鼻祖——涪翁
The Pioneer of Acupuncture——Fu Weng

涪翁（西汉末年到东汉初年），四川绵阳人，是第一位载入正史的四川医家。据《后汉书·郭玉传》记载："初，有父老不知何出，常渔钓于涪水，因号涪翁。乞食人间，见有疾者，时下针石，辄应时而效。乃著《针经》《诊脉法》传于世。"可见，涪翁隐于世间，济慈于世，医德高尚，妙手回春还分文不取，以至于自己还要乞食于人。涪翁医术高明且擅长针灸疗法，他所著的《针经》则是我国第一部针灸类专著。此后，涪翁将自己的医术传授给弟子程高，程高又传给了自己的徒弟郭玉。郭玉医术十分高明，曾任东汉和帝时太医丞，并被载入《后汉书》。

　　绵阳百姓为了纪念涪翁，明代时期在南山修建了十贤堂，南山名为涪翁山。涪翁曾经居住的渔父村还建有涪翁祠纪念堂。

　　Fu Weng (from the late Western Han Dynasty to the early Eastern Han Dynasty), a native of Mianyang city, Sichuan province, was the first Sichuan acupuncturist recorded in official history. According to *The Biography of Guo Yu in the Hou Han Shu* [*History of the Later Han Dynasty*], "Once upon a time, an old man (We do not find out where he came from originally) often went fishing in the Fujiang River, so people called him Fu Weng (old man Fu), who earned his living by begging. If he met someone with a disease, he often treated them using acupuncture, which was immediately effective. He wrote *Zhen Jing* [*Acupuncture Classic*] and *Zhen Mai Fa* [*Method of Pulse Diagnosis*] to pass down his knowledge to posterity."*Zhen Jing* was the first book about acupuncture in China. However, Fu Weng was not interested in being involved in public life. As an acupuncturist of good character, he helped others, expecting nothing in return, but chose to beg for food. He was a skilled doctor who specialised in acupuncture. Fu Weng later taught his medical skills to his disciple Cheng Gao, who passed them on to his own disciple Guo Yu. As a highly skilled doctor, Guo Yu became a medical official during the reign of the He Emperor of the Eastern Han Dynasty and was listed in the *Hou Han Shu* [*History of the Later Han Dynasty*].

To commemorate Fu Weng, the people of Mianyang built the Hall of Ten Sages on Nanshan Mountain (also called Fu Weng Mountain) during the Ming Dynasty. There is also a Fu Weng Ancestral Hall in the village where he once lived.

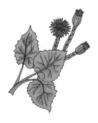

第三章

古老的中药与现代科技

Section Three Traditioanl Chinese Medicine and Modern Technology

中药的使用历史记载可追溯到上古时期的《神农本草经》，按其药性分为上、中、下三品，植物、动物和矿物皆可入药。自古以来，很多药物的发现与应用有着独特而神秘的传奇色彩，随着科学技术的发展，现代中药已成为人类防病治病的重要手段。

The historical record of the use of Chinese herbals can be traced back to the ancient *Shen Nong Ben Cao Jing* [*Shen Nong's Classic of Materia Medica*]. According to their properties, Chinese herbs are divided into three categories: top-grade, middle-grade, and inferior-grade. However, plants, animals, and minerals can all be used in traditional medicine. Since ancient times, the discovery and application of many drugs have been the subjects of unique and wonderful legends. With the development of science and technology, to this day, modern Chinese medicine remains an important approach to human disease prevention and treatment.

屠呦呦与青蒿素
Tu Youyou and Artemisinin

　　中国中医科学院著名研究员屠呦呦的名字，源自于《诗经》中的名句"呦呦鹿鸣，食野之蒿"。这个富有诗意和神秘色彩的名字，似乎预言了屠呦呦会与青蒿结下不解之缘。屠呦呦小时候机缘巧合地认识了一位老中医，这位老中医算是屠呦呦的启蒙人。他教会屠呦呦辨认最常见的中草药，使她懂得这些草药可以治病救人，普济众生。她曾听说这位老中医用中草药治疗了被毒蛇咬伤的小朋友、身患伤寒的老爷爷，于是研究中草药的种子便开始在屠呦呦的心里萌芽。从此她立志要当一位采药人，让家人远离病痛。带着儿时的梦想，屠呦呦最终成了中医科学院的科研人员。如同神农尝百草一样，一丝不苟的她也总是会在实验室里口尝身试所研究的草药。

Tu Youyou, a famous researcher at the China Academy of Chinese Medical Science, took her name from a quote in *Shi Jing* [*The Book of Songs*]: "With pleased 'youyou' sounds, the deer call to one another, eating the southernwood in the fields." This poetic and mysterious name seemed to predict that Tu Youyou would become attached to Artemisia annua. When Tu Youyou was a child, she met an old herbalist by chance. The herbalist taught her how to identify the most common Chinese herbs and enabled her to understand that such ordinary herbs may have magic powers to cure certain diseases and save lives. Tu Youyou also heard that the herbalist had used Chinese herbs to treat a child bitten by a venomous snake and cure a grandfather suffering from typhoid fever. The seeds of Chinese herbal medicine began to sprout in Tu Youyou's heart. She decided to be a herb gatherer when she grew up to keep her family free from illness. With her childhood dream in mind, Tu Youyou eventually became a researcher at the Academy of Chinese Medical Sciences. Just as Shen Nong tasted various kinds of herbs, Tu Youyou, who was serious and cautious, always experimented personally with herbs in the laboratory.

疟疾，民间俗称"打摆子"，这种病是由于人体感染疟原虫引起，能快速传播并能引发大规模的流行。根据记载，疟疾曾经在世界上102个国家和地区流行，也曾经是军队行动的无形杀手。20世纪60年代越南战争时期，正是疟疾再次肆虐东南亚的时期，1961—1967年越南军队中患疟疾的病员人数远远超过了战争伤员的人数。应越南要求，中共中央决定紧急援助。我国科学技术委员会和中国人民解放军总后勤部召开了"疟疾防治药物研究工作协作会议"，部署了代号为"523"的任务，1969年，中国中医研究院参与其中。当时39岁的屠呦呦因扎实的中西医知识和公认的科研能力被任命为课题组组长。这也是该任务取得重大进展的开始。

Malaria, popularly known in China as "Da Bai Zi" (suffering from malaria), is a mosquito-borne infectious disease caused by the malaria parasite, which can spread rapidly and cause large-scale epidemics. According to the archives, malaria was once endemic in 102 countries and regions worldwide, and it was once an invisible killer of those engaged in military operations. During the Vietnam War of the 1960s, malaria once again hit Southeast Asia.

The number of malaria patients was far higher than the number of war casualties caused by the war between 1961 and 1967. At the request of Vietnam, the Central Committee of the Communist Party of China (CPC) decided to provide emergency assistance. Therefore, the State Science and Technology Commission and the General Logistics Department of the Chinese People's Liberation Army held a collaboration meeting to discuss malaria drug research,deploying the mission code-named "523". In 1969, the China Academy of Traditional Chinese Medicine joined the mission. Tu Youyou, who was 39, at the time, was appointed head of the research group because of her solid knowledge of Chinese and Western medicine, as well as her renowned scientific research ability. It was also the beginning of significant progress for the mission.

屠呦呦肩负着艰巨的任务，大量翻阅历代医籍，查阅群众献方，请教老中医专家，并带着药箱，走进了中国南方丛林地带的疟疾高发区，走访和检查着不同年龄层的疟疾患者，采集实验数据。呦呦在古籍《肘后备急方》的启迪下，筛选出了一种普通而古老的菊科植物——青蒿。在这里不得不提到给予呦呦启迪的重要书籍《肘后备急方》，此书为东晋医家葛洪所著，是我国第一部急救专著，其中记载了青蒿治疗疟疾，即民间称之为"打摆子"的疾病。

Burdened with this arduous task, Tu Youyou read numerous medical books from past dynasties, studied prescriptions offered by the masses, and consulted elderly TCM experts. Carrying a medicine kit, she visited a high-incidence area of malaria in the jungle of southern China to examine malaria patients of different ages and collect experimental data. Inspired by *Zhou Hou Bei Ji Fang* [*A Handbook of Prescriptions for Emergencies*], Youyou selected a common and ancient composite plant, Artemisia annua. It is necessary to mention the importance of *Zhou Hou Bei Ji Fang* in giving Youyou enlightenment. This book, written by the physician Ge Hong during the Eastern Jin Dynasty, is China's first treatise on emergency treatment. It records the treatment of malaria using Artemisia annua.

在实验室里，屠呦呦带领团队努力提取青蒿素作为抗疟药品。试验虽经历了一次又一次的失败，可是屠呦呦反复思考分析原因，并告诉自己不要放弃。终于，她受到《肘后备急方》中"青蒿一握，以水二升渍，绞取汁，尽服之"的启示，开创了低温提取的方法。1971年10月4日是一个特别的日子，呦呦和她的团队终于在第191次试验中成功分离出抗疟特效药物青蒿素。为证明本次试验中的青蒿提取物是安全的，呦呦和团队又充当了"小白鼠"，终于在1972年11月提取分离出后来经鼠疟试验证明显效的青蒿素晶体。此后青蒿素被用在疫区进行临床验证，成功挽救了非洲肯尼亚疫区的一位孕妇，创造了世界奇迹。青蒿素制成的新药"科泰新"也被世界公认为抗疟药物历史性的突破，一举成为我国第一个原始创新药物，并在临床中挽救了大量疟疾患者，尤其是发展中国家数百万疟疾患者的生命。

Tu Youyou and her team were working to extract artemisinin as a malaria drug. The experiment failed again and again, but Tu Youyou did not give up. Instead, she repeatedly analysed the reasons for the failure and told herself not to give up. Finally, Tu Youyou was inspired by a passage in *Zhou Hou Bei Ji Fang* —"Soak a handful of Artemisia annua in two litres of water, grind until it becomes juice and take it"—and created a low-temperature extraction method. Youyou and her team finally isolated artemisinin, an effective antimalarial drug, in the 191st trial on October 4, 1971. To prove the Artemisia annua extract from this experiment was safe, Youyou and her team conducted clinical trials on themselves as guinea pigs. Finally, they extracted and isolated artemisinin crystals, which proved to be effective in tests on actual laboratory mice in November 1972. Since then, artemisinin has been used for clinical verification in epidemiology and successfully saved a pregnant woman in the epidemic area of Kenya, Africa, creating a global miracle. Ke Tai Xin (Dihydroartemisinin tablets), a new drug made from artemisinin, has also been recognised as a historic breakthrough in antimalarial medicine. It became the first innovative drug to originate from China and saved millions of malaria patients in clinical practice, especially in developing countries.

由于成功提取青蒿素并应用于临床治疗取得成就，2011 年，屠呦呦获得美国拉斯克医学奖；2015 年 10 月又获得诺贝尔生理学或医学奖。2019 年，屠呦呦被授予共和国勋章，同年 10 月荣获联合国教科文 – 赤道几内亚国际生命科学研究奖。屠呦呦和青蒿这株神奇的绿色小草改变了世界，也是中国传统医学贡献给世界的宝贵礼物。

For the successful extraction and clinical application of artemisinin, Tu Youyou received the 2011 Lasker Medical Research Awards and the 2015 Nobel Prize in Physiology or Medicine. She was also awarded the Medal of the Republic in 2019 and the UNESCO-Equatorial Guinea International Prize for Research in the Life Sciences in October of the same year. Tu Youyou, along with Artemisia annua, the magical green grass, changed the world. They precious gifts that traditional Chinese medicine has contributed to the world.

毒药砒霜与白血病
Arsenic Trioxide Poison and Leukaemia

传统中药砒石经火煅制后有大毒，这就是人们常说的毒药砒霜。据《本草纲目》记载，砒霜有去腐生肌、枯痔杀虫之功效，其主要化学成分为三氧化二砷（As_2O_3）。20 世纪 70 年代，中国有一位既学传统中医，又学现代医学的医生张亭栋，通过临床研究发现这种有效成分为三氧化二砷的砒霜单独使用，可以治疗白血病，这种显著的抗肿瘤功效真是令人匪夷所思。

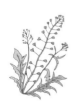

After being calcined by fire, the arsenolite used in traditional Chinese medicine becomes deadly and is commonly referred to as the poison arsenic trioxide. According to *Ben Cao Gang Mu* [*Compendium of Materia Medica*], its benefits include removing necrotic tissue and promoting granulation, destroying haemorrhoids, and killing insects. Its primary chemical constituent is arsenic trioxide (As_2O_3). Through a clinical study in the 1970s, Zhang Tingdong, a Chinese physician who had studied both traditional Chinese and Western medicine, discovered that arsenic trioxide can be used to treat leukaemia. This unique anti-tumour activity had been inconceivable.

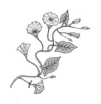

后来，中国前卫生部长陈竺院士的团队在《科学》杂志发表论文，发现三氧化二砷能够特异地结合在融合蛋白的早幼粒细胞白血病基因(PML)部分，抑制它的功能，导致癌细胞死亡，由此阐明了砒霜治疗急性早幼粒细胞白血病的机理。我国著名内科血液学专家王振义院士在国际上率先提出了应用全反式维甲酸诱导分化治疗急性早幼粒细胞白血病（APL）的"上海方案"。

Subsequently, former Minister of Health of China Chen Zhu and his colleagues published a manuscript in the journal *Science*, stating that arsenic trioxide can combine with the promyelocytic leukaemia (PML) portion of the fusion protein to disrupt its activity and kill cancer cells. Thus, the mechanism by which arsenic trioxide affects myeloid leukaemia was clarified. The "Shanghai Protocol" for treating acute promyelocytic leukaemia (APL) with all-trans retinoic acid to induce differentiation was proposed by another academician, Wang Zhenyi, a renowned Chinese haematologist specialising in internal medicine.

　　两位中国科学家在国际上首创应用全反式维甲酸和三氧化二砷联合靶向治疗初发急性早幼粒细胞白血病的患者，这类患者的 5 年无病生存率约从 25% 跃升至 95%，使其成为第一种可被治愈的急性髓系白血病。他们也因此获得了第七届圣捷尔吉癌症研究创新成就奖，该项奖是迄今为止世界在癌症研究方面的最高嘉奖，用于表彰在癌症研究中取得突出贡献的科学家。

Two Chinese researchers have pioneered a targeted therapy for newly diagnosed APL patients that uses all-trans retinoic acid in combination with arsenic trioxide. The five-year disease-free survival rate increased from approximately 25% to approximately 95%, making APL the first treatable acute myeloid leukaemia. The authors received the Seventh Szent-Gyorgyi Prize for Progress in Cancer Research, the world's most prestigious award for scientists who have made remarkable contributions to cancer research.

值得一提的是，上述全反式维甲酸也是一个针对 PML–RARα 的天然靶向药物，它结合的是 RARα，而砒霜结合的是 PML，这两个针对 PML–RARα 融合蛋白的靶向药物，一个像手铐，一个像脚铐，同时使用，就能彻底锁死融合蛋白。这就是为什么"砒霜 + 全反式维甲酸"混合疗法对急性早幼粒细胞白血病有效率会接近 100%，这种联合靶向疗法已成为国际上治疗急性早幼粒细胞白血病的标准疗法，治疗急性早幼粒细胞白血病的靶向治疗研究也成为转化医学研究的典范。

All-trans retinoic acid is also a natural medication that targets PML-RARα by binding to RARα. Arsenic trioxide, on the other hand, binds to PML. Two drugs targeting the PML-RARα fusion protein, one like a handcuff and one like an ankle cuff, are used simultaneously to completely lock up the fusion protein. This is why the arsenic and all-trans retinoic acid combination treatment for acute promyelocytic leukaemia achieved a response of nearly 100%. In other words, the "arsenic plus all-trans retinoic acid" combination therapy was found to have a near-total success rate against acute promyelocytic leukaemia. This multimodal targeted therapy is now the standard treatment for APL around the globe. The targeted therapeutic research for APL must also serve as an example for translational medical research.

As_2O_3 治疗白血病效果良好，已被美国食品药品管理局批准用于治疗急性早幼粒细胞白血病。近年来的研究表明，As_2O_3 既能治疗血液系统肿瘤，又对其他多种实体肿瘤具有抑制作用，可以说砒霜是一种天然的靶向药物，印证了中药"以毒攻毒"的科学性以及"毒即药"的神奇疗效。

As_2O_3 has been licensed by the US Food and Drug Administration for treating acute promyelocytic leukaemia as a highly successful treatment. In recent years, As_2O_3 has been demonstrated to inhibit haematological cancers and other solid tumours. Arsenic trioxide, the natural targeted drug, arguably proves the scientificity of the "fight poison with poison" philosophy of traditional Chinese medicine and the magical therapeutic effect of "poison as medicine".

第四章

诗歌里的中医药故事

Section Four Traditional Chinese Medicine Stories in Poetry

传统医学是优秀传统文化的重要组成部分，中医药凝聚着深邃的智慧，从《诗经》开始就有许多关于中草药的描述，各朝代的诗人也留下了脍炙人口的诗词经典，成为中华优秀传统文化璀璨的明珠，世代咏传。

Traditional medicine is an important part of excellent traditional culture. Traditional Chinese medicine embodies profound wisdom. Beginning with *The Book of Songs*, there have been many descriptions of Chinese herbals. In every historical dynasty, many popular poetry classics have been written, which have become the shining pearl of Chinese excellent traditional culture, having been handed down from generation to generation.

呦呦鹿鸣，食野之蒿

The Deer Call with Joyful "Youyou" Sound, Eating the Southernwood in the Fields

中国科学家屠呦呦的名字出自《诗经·小雅·鹿鸣》。其中，"呦呦"指的是鹿鸣之声，而"蒿"则指中草药"青蒿"，也就是《肘后备急方》中记载的治疗疟疾的中药，也是屠呦呦用来提取青蒿素的原料。《诗经》里的这句话自然而然地将屠呦呦与青蒿联系在了一起，成了这位著名女科学家与青蒿素结缘的传奇佳话。

The name of the renowned Chinese scientist Tu Youyou derives from a quote in *Lu Ming · Xiao Ya · Shi Jing* [*The Book of Songs*]. "Youyou" refers to the sound of deer chirping and "Hao" refers to the Chinese herbal medicine southernwood, which is the traditional Chinese treatment for malaria recorded in *Zhou Hou Bei Ji Fang* [*A Handbook of Prescriptions for Emergencies*] and the raw material from which Tu Youyou extracted artemisinin. The sentence in *The Book of Songs naturally links* Tu Youyou with Artemisia annua, creating the legendary story of this famous female scientist's connection with artemisinin.

无独有偶，《诗经》中的"彼采艾兮，一日不见，如三岁兮"，也提到了艾草，即用于温灸的"艾蒿"。可见早在两千多年前，艾草就已经进入了人们的生活。艾草叶晾干，铡碎后制成艾绒，则可以卷制成艾灸条用于艾灸疗法。温灸疗法和针灸疗法均属于古老的中医疗法。因为艾草性属温，艾灸燃烧产生的温热之气会传递到皮肤里，协助人体温通气血、补益阳气。此外，艾灸疗法通过熏灸人体腧穴，可达到调理疾病、延年益寿的目的。

Coincidentally, Artemisia apiaceae was also referenced in *The Book of Songs* in the statement, "She goes to collect fresh Artemisia apiaceae every day. I do not see her for one day, which is analogous to a three-year separation." The herb Artemisia apiaceae, sometimes known as wormwood, can be used in moxibustion. As early as 2,000 years ago, Artemisia apiaceae was widely utilised. Moxa is made by drying and crushing Artemisia apiaceae leaves. It is then rolled and packed into moxibustion sticks for use in moxibustion therapy. Both warm moxibustion and acupuncture are considered ancient Chinese treatments. Since Artemisia apiaceae has heating properties, when it is burned, the warm flow of Qi may be transmitted to the skin, warming the body, ventilating the blood circulation, and replenishing Yang Qi. Additionally, moxibustion treatment can be used to cure illness and extend life by fumigating specific acupoints.

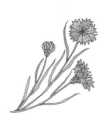

九月九日忆山东兄弟

Nostalgia for My Brothers on the Double Ninth Day

"独在异乡为异客，每逢佳节倍思亲。遥知兄弟登高处，遍插茱萸少一人。"这是唐代诗人王维（701—761年）所作的七言诗。这首诗写出了游子的思乡情怀，尤其是在农历九月初九重阳节这一天登高望远，思乡之情尤其浓烈。同时，这首诗也反映出了重阳节与中国传统文化和中医精髓密切相关的联系。重阳节，也叫重九节，《易经》将数字9定义为阳，因此得名重阳节，这也体现了中医的阴阳五行理论。同时，九为数之极，寓意大、久而长寿，因此现在也称重阳节为老人节，希望老人长寿久安。

Alone, a lonely stranger in a foreign land,

I doubly pine for kinsfolk on a holiday.

I know my brothers would, with dogwood spray in hand,

Climb up mountain and miss me so far away.

Translated by Xu Yuanchong

Wang Wei , a Tang Dynasty poet, wrote a seven-character poem conveying his homesickness when he was away from home, especially on September 9 of the lunar calendar, the Double Ninth Festival, when people climb to high points and look far into the distance. At the same time, this poem also reflects the close bond between the Double Ninth Festival and the the essence of traditional Chinese medicine in traditional Chinese culture. The Chonyang Festival is also known as the Double Ninth Festival since the number nine was designated as Yang in *Yi Jing* [*The Book of Changes*], which is in line with the Chinese medical principles of Yin-Yang and the Five Elements. It is a day to show respect to the elderly and look more closely at the lives of the older generation. It is celebrated on September 9 of the lunar calendar because, in Chinese folklore, the number nine is the largest number and a homonym of the Chinese word jiu, so the name contains the auspicious meaning of "a long and healthy life".

而在九月九重阳节插茱萸的风俗也由来已久。在晋代周处所著的《风土记》中有记载说九月九日把茱萸插在头上，就是取中药山茱萸性温、辟邪气、御初寒的功效，具体来说就是希望能通过头戴茱萸来祈求平安和避免染上瘟疫。植物茱萸通常分为山茱萸和吴茱萸，吴茱萸主要生长在现在江浙一带，是以前"吴国"的所在地产的茱萸，而山茱萸全国皆有。在本诗里，山东并非指的是今天的山东省，而是函谷关华山以东，因此其中的茱萸应该不是吴茱萸，而是山茱萸。山茱萸性温，味酸涩，补肾涩精，是著名的中成药"六味地黄丸"中的一

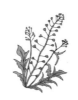

味药物。

杜甫在《九日寓蓝田崔氏庄》里也提到："明年此会知谁健，醉把茱萸仔细看。"描述了重阳团聚、饮酒、插茱萸的习俗，也暗示着茱萸可以强身健体的意思。

During the Chongyang Festival, it has long been customary to harvest and wear dogwood blossoms. This follows a traditional Chinese medicine practice intended to ward off evil and cold according to *Fengdoji* [*Feng Tu Ji*], a book written by Zhou Chu during the Jin Dynasty that focuses on documenting customs. By wearing the blossom, people were praying explicitly for peace and health, hoping to avoid any plagues. Dogwood comes in two varieties: Cornus and Evodia. Jiangsu and Zhejiang provinces, the old State of Wu, are home to most of China's Evodia plantations. Cornus, on the other hand, can be found across China. In the poem, Shandong does not refer to the province of Shandong in China but to the region east of the Hangu Passes, where the Mount Hua rises. As a result, the dogwood in the poem should be Cornus rather than Evodia. Dogwood is warm, sour, and astringent, so it can tonify the kidneys and arrest seminal emission. It is also one of the ingredients of the famous Chinese medicine "Liuwei Dihuang Pills" (Pills of six ingredients with rehmannia). Du Fu, a renowned poet also mentioned in *Nine Days Residence in Cui's Mason in Lantian*, "Because no one can foretell what will happen in the following year, why not drink while staring at the Cornus?" This statement describes the custom of drinking wine, picking Cornus, and wearing it at a family reunion during the festival, all of which serve to keep one healthy.

第五章

传统节日的中医药故事

Section Five Traditional Chinese Medicine Stories from

Traditional Festivals

中医经典《黄帝内经》奠定了中医学发展的理论基础，其中"故智者之养生也，必顺四时而适寒暑"这句话体现了"天人合一，顺应自然"的养生保健理念。一年四季中，传统历法包含的二十四节气也蕴含了丰富的保健知识。例如，"春生，夏长，秋收，冬藏"就体现了中医传统文化中顺应节气变化来调理生活方式的养生之道。2016 年 11 月，中国传统历法中的"二十四节气"被正式列入联合国教科文组织人类非物质文化遗产代表作名录。中医药文化与中华传统文化、中国民风民俗息息相关，也是中国优秀传统文化的重要组成部分。此外，中医药文化在中国传统节日中也有所体现。

Huang Di Nei Jing [*The Yellow Emperor's Inner Canon*], a classic of traditional Chinese medicine, laid the theoretical foundations for the development of TCM. The sentence "... a wise person follows the rules of four seasons to keep healthy" embodies the healthcare concept of "harmony between nature and man, conforming to nature". Among the four seasons of the year, the twenty-four solar terms of the traditional calendar contain a wealth of health knowledge. For example, "born in spring, grow in summer, harvest in autumn, and store in winter" is a way of maintaining health in traditional Chinese medicine by adapting to the changes of solar terms. In November 2016, the twenty-four solar terms of the traditional Chinese calendar were officially included in the list of representative works of the UNESCO Intangible Cultural Heritage of Humanity. Chinese medical culture is closely related to Chinese traditional culture and folklore, and it is also an important aspect of the excellent traditional culture of China. Besides, Chinese medical culture is also reflected in Chinese traditional festivals.

清明节与中医药

Qingming Festival (Tomb-Sweeping Day) and
Traditional Chinese Medicine

清明节，与春节、中秋节和端午节一起并称为中国四大传统节日。清明是冬至后的第 104 天，也是春分后第 15 天，清明节大约始于周代，起源于古代帝王将相"墓祭"之礼，已有 2500 多年的历史。正如诗中所言："清明时节雨纷纷，路上行人欲断魂"，清明节是祭祖和扫墓的日子。北宋文豪黄庭坚写下了"佳节清明桃李笑，野田荒冢自生愁"，既表达了思念故人的悲伤，又书写了踏青赏景的惬意。因此，祭祖、郊游和观光成了中国人在清明节期间的一种固定风俗。清明节也作为重要传统节日，于 2006 年被列入第一批国家级非物质文化遗产名录。

The Qingming Festival is one of the four main traditional Chinese festivals, along with the Spring Festival, the Mid-Autumn Festival, and the Dragon Boat Festival. It is the 104th day after the winter solstice and the 15th day after the spring equinox. With a history of more than 2,500 years, it began sometime in the Zhou Dynasty and originated from the ritual of "sweeping tombs and offering sacrifices to ancestors". As mentioned in the poem "A drizzling rain falls like tears on the Mourning Day; The mourner's heart is going to break on his way", the Qingming Festival is a day to worship one's ancestors and sweep tombs. Huang Tingjian, a great writer during the Northern Song Dynasty, wrote the poem "Peaches and plums are in full bloom during the Qingming Festival, while the unattended graves in the wild land make people grieve" in memory of the dead and to express the pleasure of outings and sightseeing. Thus, ancestor worship, outings, and sightseeing become fixed customs for the Chinese nation during the Qingming Festival. In 2006, the Qingming Festival, as an important traditional festival,was listed in the first batch of the National List of Intangible Cultural Heritage.

春季生机勃发，万物生长，中医认为人的机体也如此，立春以后肝气随着气温升高而逐渐旺盛，在清明之际达到最高点。若肝气过旺，会造成脾胃失调、情绪失调、气血运行不畅。于是在清明期间，中医也有独特的养生之道。清明菊是一味具有疏肝明目、清热解毒功效的中药材，正好用于治疗肝气过旺引发的疔疮痈疽、目赤肿痛、头晕目眩等病症。因此，在清明时节不妨喝一壶清明菊茶来起到保健养生的作用。

According to traditional Chinese medicine, spring is full of vigour and rapid growth, including the human body. After the beginning of spring, the Liver Qi gradually rises with the increasing external temperatures, reaching its highest point during the Qingming Festival. Excessive Qi leads to disorders of the spleen, stomach, and emotions, as well as Qi and blood deficiencies, so during the Qingming Festival, traditional Chinese medicine has a unique way to keep healthy. In traditional Chinese herbal medicine, chrysanthemum can soothe the liver, brighten the eyesight, clear away heat, and detoxify. Thus, it could be used to treat furuncles, carbuncles, red swelling and pain in the eyes, dizziness, and other diseases caused by excessive Liver Qi. Therefore, it is a good choice to drink chrysanthemum tea to prevent diseases during the Qingming Festival.

在我国江南地区，清明时节有吃青团的习俗。青团，以艾蒿和糯米为原材料制作而成。艾蒿为菊科蒿属植物，又被称为清明菜，能调理脾胃，还能利胆、抗菌除湿、消食降火，更能避邪气、驱蚊虫。人们摘取鲜嫩的艾蒿嫩芽，捣碎取汁，然后在汁水中加入糯米粉，将汁水与糯米粉拌匀，加入蔬菜馅儿或者芝麻馅儿蒸熟食用。不好消化的糯米与能调理脾胃的艾蒿两两搭配，相得益彰，堪称妙品。这就是为什么江南人一直将青团作为祭品供奉祖先的原因，清明节吃青团也已经成为民俗的一部分。

In the Jiangnan region of China, people eat Qingtuan (sweet green rice balls made with glutinous rice and mugwort) during the Qingming Festival. As mugwort belongs to Artemisia of Compositae, it is also known as a Qingming dish that can regulate the spleen and stomach, while it also good for the gallbladder. Furthermore, it resists bacteria, removes dampness, promotes digestion, clears internal heat, repels insects, and drives out evil spirits. People pick fresh mugwort leaf buds, mash them into juice, add glutinous rice flour to this green juice, and stuff the mixture with vegetable or sesame seed fillings. Therefore, the indigestible glutinous rice and the digestion-promoting mugwort are a perfect match and a delicious food. This is why the Jiangnan people give Qingtuan as an offering to their ancestors. Eating Qingtuan during the Qingming Festival has also become part of their folklore.

传说有一年清明节，太平天国的一位将领陈太平被清兵追捕，农民帮助陈太平化装成农民模样逃过了追捕并躲在了草丛里。农民回家后想给陈太平带点果腹的食物，突然他不小心摔了一跤，倒在了艾草上，双手沾满了绿色的汁水。他顿时计上心头，采了艾草回家挤出艾草的汁儿，混进糯米粉里做成了绿油油的青团，将青团滚在草地里混过了清兵的搜查，最终送到陈太平手中。陈太平吃了青团觉得又香又糯真好吃，在他逃出来之后，下令太平军学做青团以自保，于是吃青团的习俗就流传下来了。因此清明吃青团除了养生保健，更表达了人们对美好生活的期待。

Legend has it that one year during the Qingming Festival, Chen Taiping, a general of the Taiping Heavenly Kingdom, was being pursued by the Qing army. He temporarily escaped from the enemy with the help of a farmer and hid in the grass. After the farmer returned home, he thought about bringing food to Chen Taiping. He tripped accidentally and fell down onto mugwort, staining his hands with green juice. A good idea came to his mind: he picked some mugwort, brought it home to squeeze out the juice, mixed it with glutinous rice flour to make Qingtuan, and rolled the rice balls in the meadowland. The Qing army were deceived by this trick and the farmer finally brought the Qingtuan to Chen Taiping. Chen ate the Qingtuan and found it fragrant and glutinous. After he managed to escape, he ordered the Taiping army to learn how to make Qingtuan for self-protection, so the custom of eating Qingtuan was passed down. Thus, eating Qingtuan during the Qingming Festival is not only for healthcare; it also expresses the desire for a better life.

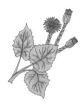

端午节与中医药
The Dragon Boat Festival and Traditional
Chinese Medicine

　　端午节是每年的农历五月初五，又名端阳节，龙舟节，也是中国首批入选世界非物质文化遗产的节日。传说端午节的起源和纪念古代爱国诗人屈原有关。屈原是战国时期楚国人，政治家，他早年受到楚怀王的信任，管内政外交大事。后来屈原被王公贵族排挤而遭到流放，在楚国的都城被秦军攻破以后，屈原出于爱国之情，自沉于汨罗江殉国。人们划着船寻觅不到屈原的踪影，就将竹筒米饭撒在江中，以防他的身体被鱼虾咬食。于是五月初五这一天，就成为端午节，竹筒米饭改为粽子，小船改为龙舟，以此纪念屈原，一代一代传下来成了中国的传统风俗。

The Dragon Boat Festival (also known as the Duanyang Festival) is held in the fifth lunar month and is the first Chinese festival to be inscribed on the World Intangible Culture Heritage list. Legend has it that the origins of the Dragon Boat Festival are linked to the commemoration of the ancient patriotic poet Qu Yuan. Qu Yuan was a native and a statesman of the State of Chu during the Warring States Period. He was trusted by King Huai of Chu to manage domestic and foreign affairs in his early years, but was later ostracised by the nobles and exiled. After the capital of Chu was occupied by the Qin army, Qu drowned himself in the Miluo River out of a sense of patriotism. People rowed out in boats to find Qu Yuan but in vain, so they scattered bamboo rice in the river to prevent his body from being bitten by fish and shrimps. The fifth day of May became the Dragon Boat Festival and people use Zongzi (rice dumplings wrapped in reeds) and dragon boats to commemorate Qu Yuan, which has become a traditional Chinese custom passed down from generation to generation.

端午节除了划龙舟、包粽子，也自然少不了中草药的身影，尤其是艾叶、菖蒲和雄黄。中医认为雄黄性温，味苦、辛，有毒，但是外用可作为解毒药治疗疥癣、虫咬等所致的皮肤病。此外雄黄还能克制蛇、蝎等百虫，有杀百毒、辟百邪的功效。因此在端午节洒点雄黄酒能起到"祈福去百病"的作用。与此同时，端午节前后，雨量增多，气温升高，蚊虫等也会顺势增多。而艾叶这种菊科植物，五月长势喜人，正如古诗所云："端午时节草萋萋，野艾茸茸淡着衣。"艾草是中医常用中草药，茎叶都含有挥发性芳香油，可以驱虫除蝇。据《本草纲目》记载"艾草性温，味辛，苦，有小毒，能温经散寒，祛湿止痒"，是灸法治病的重要药材，因此民间常有"家有三年艾，郎中不用来"的说法。此外，菖蒲也是含有挥发性芳香油的一种草药，能杀虫灭菌，它的叶子狭长犹如一把宝剑，被古人称之为水剑，寓意为斩千邪，只要端午节在门口悬挂菖蒲，邪虫毒物是不敢轻易进屋的。因此在家门口悬挂艾草和菖蒲也成了端午节的习俗之一。

In addition to activities like rowing dragon boats and wrapping Zongzi, Chinese herbal medicines, especially mugwort leaves, calamus, and realgar, are also indispensable during the Dragon Boat Festival. Chinese medicine holds that realgar is warm in nature, as well as bitter and pungent in taste. Although poisonous, it can be used externally as an antidote to scabies, insect bites, and other skin diseases. In addition, realgar is believed to drive out poisonous animals like snakes and scorpions, as well as evil spirits. Therefore, during the Dragon Boat Festival, people spread realgar wine to "eradicate diseases." At the same time, the higher rainfall and temperature around the time of the Dragon Boat Festival lead to rapidly increasing mosquito populations. Mugwort, a composite plant which grows well in May, is a common herbal treatment in traditional Chinese medicine. Its stems and leaves contain volatile aromatic oil that can repel insects and flies. As *Ben Cao Gang Mu* [*Compendium of Materia Medica*] recorded, "Mugwort is warm in nature, bitter and pungent in taste, and contains minimal toxicity, which can warm the meridian, dissipate cold, remove dampness and relieve itching". It is an important medicinal material for moxibustion treatment. Therefore, there is a saying in folklore that "three-year-old moxa grass keeps the doctor away". In addition, calamus, another herbal medicine that contains volatile aromatic oil, can kill insects and bacteria. Its long, sword-like leaves are called water swords, which symbolise cutting down all evil spirits. Thus, hanging mugwort and calamus on the door could prevent poisonous insects from entering, which is also a custom of the Dragon Boat Festival.

在端午节，民间还有将菖蒲和艾叶晒干制成香囊让小孩佩戴于胸前的习俗，此法能有效驱虫辟邪，醒神开窍，提高孩童的免疫力和增进食欲，这也是具有中医特色的"衣冠疗法"之一。菖蒲和艾草还能一起熬水用于药浴，达到预防疾病的效果。"五月五日午，天师骑艾虎。蒲剑斩百邪，鬼魅入虎口"正是描述端午节人们利用中草药治未病的预防保健方式，也是人们祈福的象征。

During the Dragon Boat Festival, dried calamus and mugwort leaves are also put into sachets for children to repel insects and exorcise evil spirits, refresh the children's minds, improve their immunity, and enhance their appetite. This is also one of the "clothing therapies" in traditional Chinese medicine. Calamus and mugwort can also be boiled together as medicinal baths to prevent disease. As the saying goes, "At noon on the fifth day of May, the Heavenly Master rode a tiger made of mugwort to cut down all the evil spirits with a sword made of calamus, and all the evil spirits were eaten by the tiger." This proverb illustrates why Chinese herbal medicine is used to cure disease and keep healthy during the Dragon Boat Festival, as well as being a symbol of blessing.

中秋节与中医药
The Mid-Autumn Festival and Traditional
Chinese Medicine

　　每年农历的八月十五是我国的传统节日中秋节。从先秦时期起，古代帝王便有春天祭日，秋天祭月的传统。"中秋"一词最早见于《周礼》，其中有"夜明，祭月也"的记载。而中秋正式成为重要的民俗节日，始于唐朝。中秋节除了有吃月饼的习俗外，还会饮桂花酒。根据《本草汇言》记载，桂花，散冷气，消瘀血，止肠风血痢。桂花酒是我国最具特色的传统酒之一，每逢八月，金桂飘香，既是赏桂的最佳季节，又是品桂花酒的时节。桂花酒应时养生，能祛除胃寒、胃痛，温而不燥，温润脾胃，对缓解秋燥也有一定作用。

The Mid-Autumn Festival, which is on the 15th day of August each year according to the lunar calendar, has also been a traditional Chinese festival since ancient times. Since the Pre-Qin Period, the ancient emperors followed the tradition of offering sacrifices to the sun in spring and to the moon in autumn. The term "Mid-Autumn" first appeared in *Zhou Li* [*Rites of the Zhou*], which recorded that "When it is bright at night, it is time to offer sacrifices to the moon." The Mid-Autumn Festival officially became an important folk festival in the Tang Dynasty. People usually eat mooncakes and drink sweet-scented osmanthus-flavoured wine during this festival. According to *Ben Cao Hui Yan* [*Collection of Materia Medica*], osmanthus flowers can dissipate chills, eliminate congestion, and stop diarrhoea and hemafecia caused by gastrointestinal disorders. Osmanthus wine is one of the most distinctive traditional wines in China. With the fragrance of osmanthus all around, August is the best season to not only enjoy osmanthus but also taste osmanthus wine. As osmanthus wine is warm but not dry, it can dispel stomach cold, ease aches, warm the spleen and stomach, and relieve dry heat in autumn.

中秋节赏月、吃月饼和石榴也是中秋节传统习俗。我们先来看看赏月的习俗。大诗人李白曾经在《把酒问月》中写下"白兔捣药秋复春，嫦娥孤栖与谁邻"的诗句，这首诗提到了玉兔在月宫中捣药的传说。汉乐府《董逃行》提到了月宫中的兔子浑身洁白，被称为玉兔，传说玉兔一直在月宫中用玉杵捣药，制成的蛤蟆丸服用后可长生不老。久而久之，玉兔也成了月亮的代名词。而中秋月圆，象征家庭团团圆圆，吃月饼也就是取一个团圆之意。同时，月饼中包含的松仁、核桃仁、芝麻等大多为药食同源的食物，不仅美味还能保健养生。而中秋时节的石榴则是张骞出使西域从中亚引入的水果，其入药最早记载于南北朝时期陶弘景的《名医别录》，"药家用酸者""入药惟根壳而已""子为服食者所忌"，也就是说，石榴入药的部分是干燥的果皮。其主要功效是涩肠止泻、收敛止血，用于治疗长时间腹泻。

Enjoying the full moon, as well as eating mooncakes and pomegranates, are also traditional Mid-Autumn Festival customs. Let's look at the custom of enjoying the full moon.

The great poet Li Bai once mentioned the legend of the jade rabbit mashing medicine in the moon palace in the poem *Ba Jiu Wen Yue* [*Drinking by Moonlight*]: "On the moon, the white rabbit pounds medicine from autumn to spring, and Chang'e lives alone, accompanied by nobody." According to *Dong Tao Xing* [*The Escape of Dong Zhuo*], a *Yuefu* song from the Han Dynasty, the rabbit in the moon palace is completely white, so it is called the Jade Rabbit. It is said that the Jade Rabbit has been pounding medicine with a jade pestle in the moon palace, and a pill made of toads can allow people to achieve immortality after taking it. As time passed, the Jade Rabbit became synonymous with the moon. Besides the full moon, mooncakes also symbolise reunion during the Mid-Autumn Festival. Furthermore, pine kernels, walnut kernels, and sesame seeds contained in mooncakes can also be used as medicine, so they are not only delicious but also healthy. The pomegranate eaten during the Mid-Autumn Festival is a fruit introduced from Central Asia by the West Han Dynasty ambassador Zhang Qian following his mission to the West. The earliest record of applying pomegranate as a kind of Chinese herb can be found in the ancient medical book known as *Ming Yi Bie Lu*[*Miscellaneous Records of Famous Physicians*], which was compiled by Tao Hongjing during the Southern and Northern Dynasties. As recorded in the text, the main function of dried pomegranate skin is to astringe the intestines to relieve diarrhoea and stop intestinal bleeding caused by prolonged diarrhoea.

因此，在传统的中秋佳节，以月之圆预示家庭圆满，而饮桂花酒、食月饼和石榴的风俗，也无时无刻不体现着中医药在传统文化中的地位。

Therefore, according to the traditions of the Mid-Autumn Festival, the full moon indicates the reunion of the family, while the customs of drinking osmanthus wine and eating mooncakes and pomegranates also reflect the status of traditional Chinese medical culture in traditional culture.

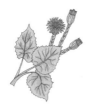

参考文献

Bibliography

［1］McCulloch D, Brown C, Iland H. Retinoic acid and arsenic trioxide in the treatment of acute promyelocytic leukemia: current perspectives[J]. Onco Targets Ther, 2017, 10:1585–1601.

［2］Swindell EP, Hankins PL, Chen H, et al. Anticancer activity of small–molecule and nanoparticulate arsenic（Ⅲ）complexes[J]. Inorg Chem, 2013, 52(21):12292–12304.

［3］Emadi A, Gore SD. Arsenic trioxide – An old drug rediscovered [J].Blood Rev, 2010, 24(4–5): 191.

［4］黄银兰 . 针灸的故事 [M]. 北京：中国中医药出版社，2020.

［5］赵宪庆 . 历史名人故事——扁鹊 [M]. 安徽：安徽美术出版社，2020.

［6］周峰 . 中医药文化故事：汉英对照 [M]. 重庆：重庆大学出版，2019.

［7］绵阳地方志办公室 . 绵阳名人 [M]. 成都：四川大学出版社，2019.

［8］金虹 . 中医药历史文化基础 [M]. 北京：中国中医药出版

社，2018.

［9］高剑坤，王谷，吴静蓉，等．靶向抗癌治疗存在的问题及
发展方向 [J]. 医学争鸣， 2018, 9 (6):12–16.

［10］中国中医科学院．屠呦呦传 [M]. 人民出版社，2018.

［11］陈子杰．中医药文化校园普及读本（三年级上册）[M].
北京：人民卫生出版社，2018.

［12］李峰．中医药文化校园普及读本（四年级上册）[M]. 北
京：人民卫生出版社，2018.

［13］钱会南．中医药文化校园普及读本（五年级上册）[M].
北京：人民卫生出版社，2018.

［14］于天源．中医药文化校园普及读本（六年级上册）[M].
北京：人民卫生出版社，2018.

［15］阚湘苓，国华，李淳．杏林初探寻中医 [M]. 北京：中医
古籍出版社，2018.

［16］李德杏，阚湘苓，李淳．中医四大名著 [M]. 北京：中医
古籍出版社，2018.

［17］王蕾，阚湘苓，李淳．医家医著学中医 [M]. 北京：中医
古籍出版社，2018.

［18］田露，阚湘苓，李淳．诗情画意品中医 [M]. 北京：中医
古籍出版社，2018.

［19］徐鲁．神奇的小草 [M]. 北京：中国少年儿童出版社，
2018.

［20］木头人儿童创想中心．上下五千年 [M]. 北京：煤炭工业
出版社，2017.

［21］张伯礼，陈传宏．中药现代化二十年[M].上海：上海科学技术出版社，2016.

［22］饶毅，张大庆，黎润红．呦呦有蒿——屠呦呦与青蒿素[M].北京：中国科学技术出版社，2015.

［23］炎继明．中国古典诗歌与中医药文化[M].西安：西安交通大学出版，2015.

［24］陈沫金．针灸的故事[M].太原：山西科学技术出版社，2014.

［25］曲黎敏．中医与传统文化[M].北京：人民卫生出版社，2009.